IVF
Are you effing *kidding* me?

aly's books
Your Book
Our Mission

Jen Lloyd

Illustrated by Matt Larkin

IVF – Are You Effing Kidding Me?

First Edition 2017
Published by Aly's Books

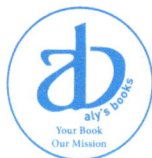

www.alysbooks.com

Edited by Sue McGregor and Irrefutable Proof
Designed by Simone Hill

ISBN: 978-0-6480017-7-5

Your journey and the path you take are yours and yours alone. It feels different and will affect you in your own way. Remember this when others tell you about their IVF journeys. This is my story and my journey, and I hope that in sharing it with you that it can help you in some small way.

Xx Jen

Let's Laugh Together

They say *laughter* is the best medicine, so hopefully my humorous take on a subject not necessarily openly spoken about or understood may help you on your own journey, or as a support person, partner, friend or family member of someone on the roller coaster of IVF, to better understand how to help! I'm not a doctor or a psychologist, but I sure know that laughing helped me. So strap yourself in for the brutal truth; a somewhat uncomfortable and at times totally inappropriate look at my IVF journey. I hope that it will give you some 'ah hah' moments, or at least a tear or two from *laughter,* and maybe make your journey just a little easier to know you are not alone in those *'batshit crazy'* moments. I'm with you and it's okay. You are doing the best you can and nobody has noticed that *eye twitch* you have going on or those giant long *chin hairs* glistening in the sun!

My Journey

My *journey* is my own and only mine, so yours may be a much simpler and more successful one – I certainly hope it is! So, how did I end up here? After all of those years on the pill you finally decide it's time to stop crossing your fingers hoping you're not pregnant and start peeing on a stick, hoping like hell it's a positive result... Well unfortunately it just wasn't that simple for me.

I didn't meet Dave until I was 36. I still felt like I was 23, but in IVF terms *I was getting old.* Now, it wasn't that I hadn't wanted children, I had since as far back as I could remember, but I just hadn't met anyone good enough to do that with, and I'm still comfortable that I never bred with any of the cheaters, con artists, gamblers and various losers I dated for years. My dad and my best mate Adam will tell you, there sure were some winners... not! (Oh, there were some good blokes in there, too, but just not right for me). I remember when I told my dad I was seeing Dave, his first question was, "Does he have a car?" When I told him that he did, his response was, "Well that's a step up from the last few!"

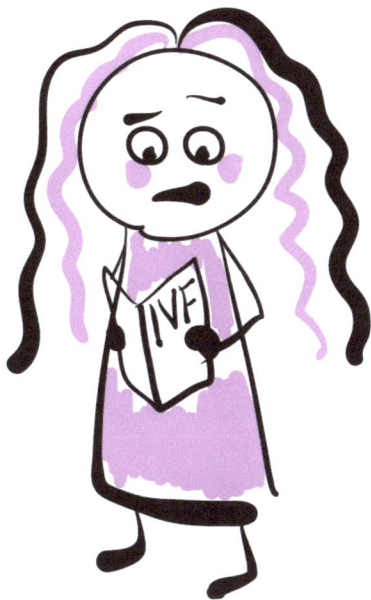

So here I was, madly in love, and in no time Dave and I were married and I had scored the two most amazing 'little people' (step-children) you could dream of! We had a trip to Europe, I came off the pill, and then the next trip was to the doctor. There were many more specialist trips after that. This was where it all began. As I tap away at this I'm 40 plus a few months (I'm telling you this because who knows when I'll get this to print, if ever!). So, five egg collections later, four failed embryo transfers and every IVF drug under the sun, including embryo glue (yes there is such a product!) and I'm still on my *journey* waiting for the test results on my one lonely embryo, waiting to see if it's 'normal'. All of my life I have never considered myself normal, always just a little different and happy to be so, but right now I damn well hope like hell that our *'Frosty'* is normal!

Where to start? The first internal ultrasound.

For years, Adam called me a *prude* because I was always 'clothes on' in public and never liked going to doctors' appointments, having successfully avoided pap smears for way too long! Yet here I was, *legs up in the air,* and some poor nurse telling me she needed to get the specialist because she couldn't insert the device properly as apparently my cervix sat forward – news to me! But what nearly pushed me over the edge was when the specialist had his face so *close to my bits* his hair was tickling my thigh! My husband Dave was in deep shock too, and as we giggled at the amount of lube applied to the device, I knew I had the right partners for my IVF journey... Dave and *laughter!*

And that is what IVF is, a journey... an *effing tough journey* that is full of needles, patches, tablets, pessaries (affectionately called rockets – I hated those most of all) and the weirdest side effects you could ever imagine. But why am I telling you this? Because *laughter* got me through it, and I hope by reading this book, you too will laugh and cry. In the moments that the pain is overwhelming and you feel like you can't breathe, here I am to remind you that you will be okay and *you are not alone!* If you are the support partner, family or friend, then I hope this book will shed some light on the journey in order to make yours that little bit easier. Dave and I have survived, and in fact become closer, but for many couples IVF is a game changer and relationship breaker, so hopefully our story will help you with yours and give you a good laugh, even if it's a little cringe-worthy at times!

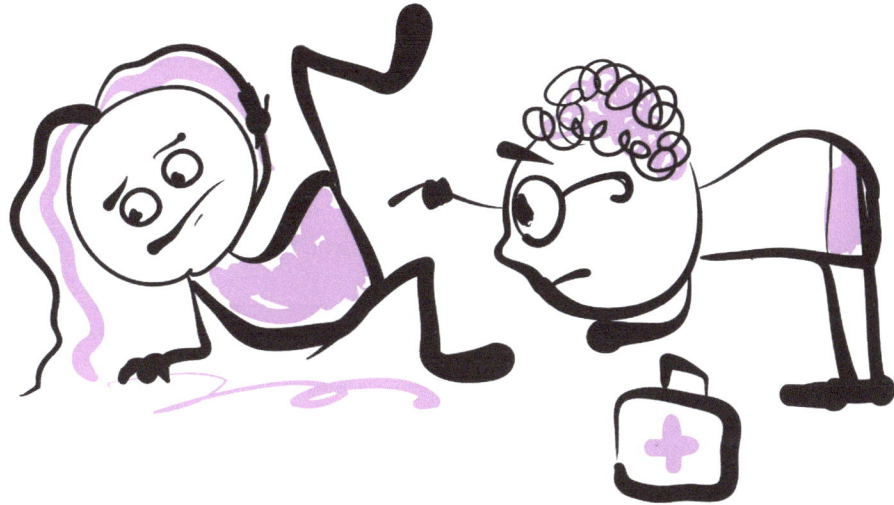

Batshit Crazy Lady

I often refer to *batshit crazy* during this book, so how did I know when I was *batshit crazy?*

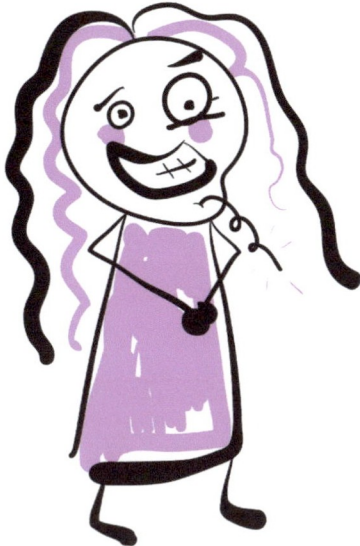

Well the eye twitching and fast growing chin hair were right up there, but it was the desire to *get on the horn*. Get on the horn you say? Yep, the car horn. All of a sudden I was tooting everyone, sticking my finger up, and I'd be sitting on Queens Road, two minutes from my office thinking, 'so the steroids have kicked in!' This type of self-awareness does help to put things in perspective and lets you know that you are reacting in a different way than you usually would. This is the best time to check in with yourself before making major decisions or before you lose your cool. Maybe write the email and then give yourself some time and review it later before sending, or ask someone you trust to let you know if you are on track with your decisions.

Clearly I love the term *batshit crazy,* so here is the urban dictionary definition:

> *"A person who is batshit crazy is certifiably nuts. The phrase has origins in the old-fashioned term "bats in the belfry". Old churches had a structure at the top called a belfry, which housed the bells. Bats are extremely sensitive to sound and would never inhabit a belfry of an active church where the bell was rung frequently. Occasionally, when a church was abandoned and many years passed without the bell being rung, bats would eventually come and inhabit the belfry. So, when somebody said that an individual had "bats in the belfry" it meant that there was "nothing going on upstairs" (as in that person's brain). To be BATSHIT CRAZY is to take this even a step further. A person who is batshit crazy is so nuts that not only is their belfry full of bats, but so many bats have been there for so long that the belfry is coated in batshit. Hence, the craziest of crazy people are BATSHIT CRAZY."*

Maybe I haven't been using quite the right terminology, but it's the craziest I've ever been in my life, therefore it will always be known by me as those *'batshit crazy'* times.

1   Urban Dictionary Definition

Crying Lady

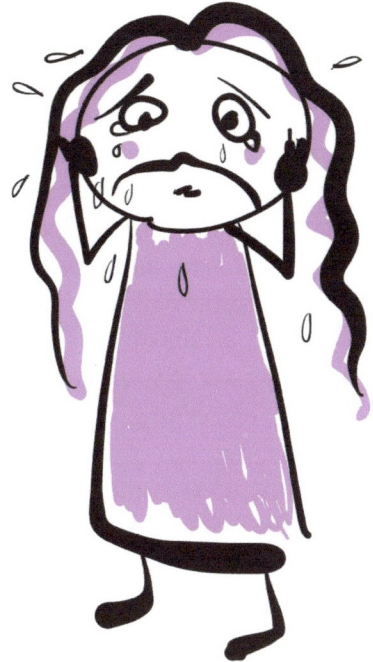

I wonder how many days, driving along the Nepean Highway, people in the next car wondered who that blonde lady singing her heart out with tears streaming down her face was. Well, it was me! Or the day I was pulled over by police, only to find out later that no I wasn't driving an unregistered car and that their equipment had made an error. They were the kindest officers when I said no it wouldn't be ok – I had an IVF appointment and here I was stuck on the side of the road with a $765 fine, an unregistered vehicle and I was absolutely *hysterical.* They were doing their best to calm this suited up lady who they'd pulled over for a routine rego check! I will always be grateful to the staff at Mercedes South Melbourne, who were prepared to drive me to my appointment if needed! Normal Jen would have managed the situation so differently, she wouldn't have cried and would have realised that they had the wrong rego, but I wasn't normal Jen. I was *five injections a day Jen,* just barely scraping through the day. Thank god Dave arrived and worked it out, whilst at the same time, the guys from Mercedes were willing to help. What a morning!

IVF Brain

Courtesy of the drugs, I have had days when I could not get my words, names or *shit together,* which is very tough for a recruiter whose memory and networking ability is how they make their money! They talk about 'preggy brain', but there is definitely a lesser known term, 'IVF brain', when your brain is so *flooded with drugs* that you don't have your normal clarity. I'm not sure anyone calls it that, but that's what I'm officially calling it and guess what, it's real and it's not your fault. There is nothing you can do. So *don't beat yourself up* if you are looking straight at someone and you've forgotten their name, or you've lost your ability to have a sense of direction (although mine was crap to start with) or you are struggling to string a sentence together. It's ok, it happened to me too, many times. I can best describe it as feeling foggy – you can't quite get clarity on anything, you want to shake your head to clear it but it doesn't happen and you quite literally feel stupid!

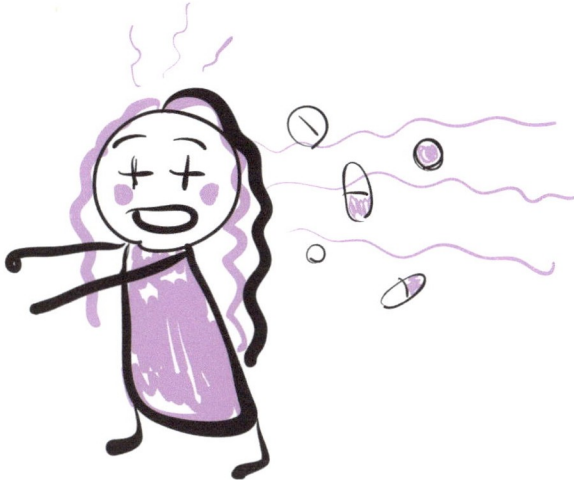

Drugs

Please don't be scared by my talk of *drugs.* Not everyone has to go through the medication I did, and many other IVF journeys aren't so complex. As described on many occasions, I had the 'trifecta of things wrong with me' and 'I must be rattling with all of those *drugs*'!

Then there was the sweet young retail girl at the pharmacy that told me she had never rung up a bill so big – really? – as I left with a Styrofoam cooler box of injections, plus a bag of scripts and another bag of multivitamins and a bill for $900! I am sure not many people can say they smashed nearly a grand in one trip to the pharmacy!

I could tick off *most of the side effects* from the many lists attached to every medication I tried. But the good news is that I never got *genital acne.* Although that didn't stop me from reminding my fabulous work colleagues that I could get them at any day, and I promised to keep them notified on any new side effects! You've got to have some fun and the side effects talk certainly freaked them out, but together we had fits of *laughter,* through the blurred vision and *chin hairs!*

Colonic Irrigation

Hmm, how does one describe it? It's seriously the weirdest sensation, not to mention bizarre, watching your *poop float* down a clear tube! Why is it clear, is it to prove it's actually doing something? Or is it our morbid fascination to see? I don't know!

Now I'm not saying anyone recommended I do it, but I thought it couldn't hurt to clean out any toxins and give my body the best chance, right? Plus I'd tried most random things people had suggested. So there I was, signed up to a three-session pack that came with tea and a body loofah – weird combo!

At session number one, whilst filling in the 'sign your life away' paperwork in case anything goes wrong, I had to write down any medications I was taking, so I did put 'currently under-going IVF treatment'. I'm not sure how someone that is trained to stick tubes up *people's bums* and makes herbal tea is an expert in all things conception, but this idiot thought she was. Off she launched about how she has a sixth sense about these things, and she could tell I was going to fall pregnant this time with IVF. But here's the thing – even though I knew her only skill was stuffing *pipes up poopers,* I was more than happy to believe her, because desperate people do desperate things. Well guess what, *poop lady?* Your sixth sense doesn't work and that is why your salon lost my business. I didn't even make the third session because I couldn't listen to her sixth sense shit. Why couldn't she just be normal and note the information, ask me if I had any questions and not interfere with my treatment? Talk about cut the crap, no pun intended! Why is it that people are compelled to *dribble shit* when someone says, "IVF"?

Never quite fitting in

This is probably the day-to-day challenge that *hurts the most!* Just not knowing where you fit. Dave's friends are mostly a bit older and have grown up children, *so I don't fit there.* My mates are all busy breeding and have two under their belt, *I don't fit there,* and my awesome colleagues are mostly in their twenties and nowhere near considering breeding, so *I don't quite fit there either.* Where is the *gang of women* that have had years of failed IVF, that get the stabbing pain when someone is rabbiting on about how tired they are because their rugrat hasn't slept properly in weeks? I'd kill to be sitting in your chair, 'living the dream' of sleepless nights, cracked nipples and way too much info about their 'poo' stories, but I'm not. You look at me and wish you had your old life back, because on Facebook my life looks so fantastic, but in reality it's not!

Not fitting in again

I've already written about not feeling like I fit in, and as Dave and I had been invited to a mutual friend's BBQ who we had only got to know recently, I thought 'this should be easy, people that don't know my journey'. My thought was, today won't hurt! I thought to myself that when they asked me if I had kids I'd simply say, "yes two, they are 15 and 11, boy and girl," I would make out I was the lucky one! They didn't need to know that they were my step-children, and they certainly didn't need to know the pain aching in my heart for my own biological child. Well, no one asked, so that was easy, but what I wasn't ready for, when hanging around with the 50s set, was talk of hysterectomies and the feeling of not being able to have any more children even though they didn't want any because they already had three grown up children that drove them nuts. My gorgeous friend gently squeezed my arm to see if I was ok with the conversation, and I was, but seriously what the hell is wrong with women, do they truly think they are only on this planet to breed? (I believe we have so much more to offer). As one talked about the sad moment when she realised that her dog was the only one able to breed in their house, post her hysterectomy, I thought, "Are you effing kidding me?" It's no surprise that I spent more time talking to the boys at that BBQ. On this occasion I was more than happy to not fit into that conversation!

Kids Parties

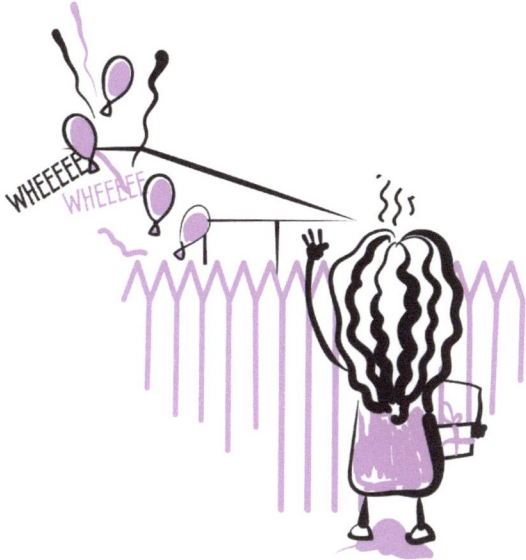

The other thing that hurts is being *excluded* from your friend's kid's party because you *don't have children.* Now, that is the worst of all. It's the biggest punch in the guts you can imagine – well it was for me! What I actually wanted was to surround myself with children, but it may not be the same for everyone. My advice is to ask the question and let the person decide. There is nothing like seeing event photos on Facebook of your friends and their kids to remind you just how shit your situation is and how you *don't fit in* anywhere anymore. I'm so grateful to some of my friends for always making *Aunty Jenny* feel so special, ensuring I am part of the parties and knowing that yes I will *eat all of the fairy bread!* I still love that stuff. If it wasn't for my niece, nephew, godson and his sister being around to make me laugh and give the hugs only a little person can, I don't know how I would have got through some of the dark days.

Disappeared

To my friends, if you didn't see me it's because *I barely left the house* other than to go to work. I had to do so many drugs at set times, and had to be home by 9pm to shoot up. Or, if you didn't have a clue and it always looked like I was having so much fun, well *Facebook can make anyone believe anything.* One St Kilda festival, it looked like Dave and I were having the best afternoon but no, I had dark glasses on because I'd cried all day with *another failed transfer,* but it was easier to look like my 'fun self' out again. Many a time I sat on *water in a beer garden,* but you'd never know, soda and lime can easily look like a gin and tonic. So don't be too quick to judge or assume what someone is going through, as what appears to be the case can be very *far from the truth.*

Being judged

This is probably the bit that *still upsets me* the most – some of the incredibly *rude* things that were said to me and said behind my back. I've always kept my *thoughts to myself* when it comes to others trying to conceive because I'm not an expert. I haven't judged other women or ever told them what they should or shouldn't do when they started trying to conceive, while they were pregnant, or what to do once they had a child. It's actually none of my business unless someone asks for my opinion, support or guidance. But why on earth do others feel like they should tell you what to do on IVF? Why is it that everyone sitting in their glasshouses of perfection think they can comment? I'm working with the best of the best at the Centre for Infertility, and they are the experts, not you. Oh, and just because on Facebook I looked like I was out having fun, you'll never know the pain I was going through, the drug regime, how many tears I'd cried that day *behind dark glasses.* A photo is a moment in time, IVF is a long slow journey of medication, fear, pain, anxiety and tears, that you wouldn't have a clue about. So, unless I ask for your opinion, which trust me I won't, keep it to yourself unless you are one the amazing women who understand, who have walked the halls of failed IVF, or for whatever reason who remain childless. Do everyone a favour and just *keep your mouth shut.*

So next time you think you should tell someone on the IVF merry-go-round what they should do, do yourself and them a favour and think about how you would feel. Not good, hey! And don't kid yourself that you're trying to be helpful – that's what IVF nurses are for – you are simply being *judgmental and opinionated!* And don't say you were worried about me, because if you were you would simply ask me how I was and if there was something you could do to help, not talk about me behind my back. My advice is don't listen, just focus on you, ignore those who don't understand and if necessary, just don't see them for a while!

Shhh, don't tell her!

Okay, so I'm still a little puzzled by this one – when people feel so uncomfortable about telling me *someone is pregnant,* they simply say nothing. Um, it's not like I'm not going to find out, they will have a baby in nine months and *I'll see it on my Facebook feed!* What do you think will happen when you tell me? I've always been an incredibly supportive friend, through the good and bad. So why would I change? Of course I'm going to be happy for that couple, maybe I might be a little bit sad on the inside that I'm not sharing the journey with them, but I'm always going to *celebrate and share their joy,* regardless of my unsuccessful attempts to have kids. Why do you think I'm now such an awful person that I can't celebrate the most important things in your life? It's not actually about how I feel, it's about you being uncomfortable, so *don't exclude me,* that only compounds the pain and isolation I already feel. You don't need to avoid me, I'm not a different person to the one I was before *IVF,* I just can't get pregnant.

First day of school

I was so excited to see all the beautiful *little people in my life* heading off for their first day of school on Facebook, and *couldn't be any prouder* of what wonderful little human beings they have grown into. But the reality of the fact that I *wouldn't have that moment* in my life cut deep, so deep that I had stabbing pain in my back, an ache in my chest and another night lying awake wondering what my life would be. Would there always be days of such sadness? Would the tears ever stop? Would I always feel left on the outside, on the fringe of conversations, being supportive and happy for others but feeling like I was slowly *dying on the inside?* I had prepared myself emotionally for certain days on the calendar that I knew would hurt, but that one came as a complete surprise.

I thought the book was finished, but then another day another page,
a little bit more of me for the world to see. I hope one day someone gets some
good from this book; I hope it helps them too.

I already know it's worth it because it's helped me deal with the pain in many ways.

Religion

Now, we were brought up Catholic, and although I still go to church at Christmas with my mum and my sister Sue, and most of our charity work is done with nuns, mainly because they are the only ones selfless enough to care for the sick and elderly - I certainly *wouldn't call myself religious.* But I did think, when I was getting more desperate for a positive outcome, that it couldn't hurt to *whack in a few prayers* to go alongside the science of IVF and Chinese medicine! So I had my mum's friend, the local nun, praying and she even announced it at mass one day, a 'prayer for Dave and Jenny on their IVF journey'. Not quite what I expected my mum to tell me after she'd been at church that day, but all the same very sweet!

On a trip to Vietnam for the charity, Sue and I were visiting the elderly women's shelter run by the Mother Teresa order of nuns, and they had large statues of Mother Teresa around the grounds. Sue convinced me (I'm still not sure if she was conning me just to make me look silly, given she is the older sister and did play some great tricks on me as a kid!) that you are supposed to *kiss the feet* of the statues, so there I was running around the grounds *kissing statues* and touching anything religious I could *for good luck.*

I can only imagine, judging by the looks on their faces, what the nuns thought the two of us were up to. Oh, and the same thing happened at a Buddhist temple. *Desperate times* call for *desperate measures,* and I was happy to give anything a go!

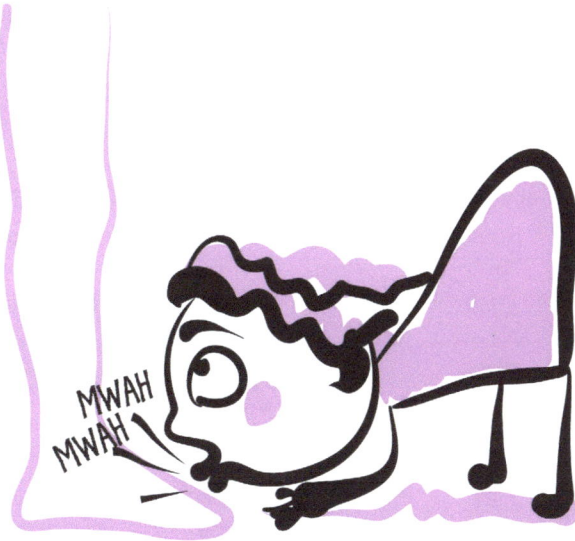

Why is it that I make you feel uncomfortable when I say I'm barren?

After years of lying or *mumbling some bullshit* when I met a woman for the first time at an event and the first question she asked was whether I had children, I just got jack of it and one day said, *"I'm barren"*. A look of horror crossed her face. Honestly ladies, we don't have to have children to have achieved something and I shouldn't have to *lie to your dumb question, to stop you from feeling uncomfortable.* I know many great women, some mums, some not, who have achieved incredible things and aren't defined by having kids, so please remember a time before you had kids when that wasn't your opening question when you met someone new. No wonder I prefer to spend time with guys, no guy has ever asked me first off at a party if I had kids!

Here are some *helpful questions* (that's the recruiter in me) that will help you connect with someone and not risk insulting them at the very same time!

How do you know the party host?

What brought you to this event?

How has your week been?

Great conversation starters, which will quickly give some insight into the other woman's life, *without making her feel like a failure* if she doesn't have children.

When I was asked at a kid's party if I had children I responded with, "yes, two step-children." Then I was asked if it was better to have stepchildren or have my own children? WTF – how would I know? *I'm barren, my bits don't work, I can't have children...* were the thoughts that came into my head, but of course I never said those out loud. I replied that my kids came with the ability to wipe their own butts, so I guess that's a positive. *Seriously ladies,* think about what comes out of your mouth. That one was a ripper but as usual, to hide my pain, I found a way to address the issue *with humour!*

You could have a miracle?

Trust me if this ever works, it won't be a miracle. It will be the work of the most amazing scientists, researchers, specialists and nurses who have worked tirelessly to help women like myself conceive. *I sit in the hands of science* as they tweak the drugs I am on to try to give me the child that *I want so badly.* There is no shining light; there is no miracle, just a *glimmer of hope* that this time, whatever I'm taking and whatever tests or surgery I need, it works.

Advice

I will have one rant and one rant only (but that may change further in to the book into many rants!)

The advice, oh the advice. Everyone has a *miracle IVF story* and as I would kindly say that can't happen for me, I'd get the "You never know dear". I wanted to scream, "I do know!!" I know Dave and I share a rare chromosome that makes my body reject the embryo, so thank you for your advice that spirulina will change everything. Or on that rare occasion when you see me out because I don't get out much when I'm up to my eye balls in preparation injections and need to be home by 9pm to shoot up, you decide you will share your opinion that I really shouldn't have that glass of wine – what would you know? You aren't exactly a picture of health, but you've been lucky enough to conceive naturally! Do you have a clue what I'm going through or how much I've changed my life to try to get pregnant and share the joy that has come so easily to you? But I say nothing, I have learned to *just smile* instead of screaming at them, "My bits don't work and you're not a fucking specialist and spirulina isn't going to change that!"

If you have never had to consider IVF but are supporting someone that is, please *think before you open your mouth* and don't say something stupid or quote something that you saw on *A Current Affair*, please! The best thing you can do is listen, give them a hug and keep your opinions and miracle stories to yourself. Oh, and if a celebrity gets pregnant in their late 40s, it's not their own egg, so yes, it's a miracle but it's a scientific miracle. I am old in IVF terms, so please don't tell me I'm not.

Rant done, lesson learnt – only surround yourself with people that offer support that makes you feel good, and only you can decide what you need.

As I say this, I still cringe at some of the things I too remember saying to friends that did IVF before me...

The IVF Badge

I don't understand it, but it appears that the years someone spends journeying through IVF are worn as a badge. Well you can *stick your badge.* I don't want to be on this merry-go-round for years, and I sure as hell wish I was like some of my lucky girlfriends that got drunk, forgot to use protection and wound up pregnant to the love of their life! One of my friends describes her first born as the best accident – a curry and a few beers!

So, here's the deal. My three years has been bloody awful from all the drugs, the additional hair, crazy arse mood swings and tears at any random moment. On a positive note, *the badge I wear* is not that I have toughed it out, but that I have the most amazing partner. Through this experience we have become better friends, and learned how to deal with each other (keeping in mind we are both Taureans and Alpha and therefore aren't backwards in sharing our opinions – we can have a damn good argument when needed).

I have also learnt who my real friends are, the ones that I can turn to in a crisis, and learned to recognise the ones that suck the life out of me. So ladies, don't compete over how long you have been stuck in this hell, *celebrate what you have gained.* For me, it's closer relationships and a better understanding of myself, and although I knew I was always resilient because I've worked in recruitment, I didn't know I was bullet proof until now! Oh, and please don't tell me about the person who finally after seven years of IVF got pregnant because I sure as shit don't want to be doing this for another 4 years. That story doesn't make me feel any better, when I'm barely able to handle the drugs on a day-to-day basis. I now know a miracle won't happen for me, scientifically it just can't!

Positive Highlights

I think it's important to *share some positivity* at this moment so you don't put the book down and run a mile. IVF Nurse – the description in the Oxford Dictionary should read *'the most caring, considerate person you will ever meet'*. I have met some of the most amazing practitioners along this journey, possibly way too many that got a little close to my lady parts for my liking but hey, you stop caring after a while and move from a well-groomed woo-woo to 70s bush and let it go!

One of the most amazing staff members was the nurse that did my internal ultrasound when I was checking the size of my follicles, in preparation for egg collection in the early days. The news wasn't great that day, as my left ovary hadn't decided to come to the party after all the drugs, and in her efforts to cheer me up she sang us her IVF song to the tune of the song from 'Frozen' (insert tune in your mind) – "is it pink, is it blue, is there one, is there two". Dave and I were in hysterics as she did the dance movements to match, all whilst conducting an internal ultrasound! Just amazing!

And I have to mention the pre-op nurse who holds your hand in those sweet seconds as the drugs kick in and you fall into a deep sleep for the procedure (those seconds were my favourite part of this entire journey). *To the nurses* that hold your hand and make you a cuppa in recovery, *you are truly special women!* Then there was my favourite blood test nurse who would distract me by telling me stories of his life growing up in Afghanistan! *You guys are incredible.*

Try to Laugh

You could literally guarantee that if there was a public holiday, I was due for a transfer or collection. So many plans shattered, or I would be doing a transfer whilst Dave was interstate with the kids – not the normal method for making a baby, husband and wifey in different states! I'll never forget the look of surprise and horror on the specialist's face the first time Dave came to a transfer with me. We'd never met her before, so she didn't know what she was in for with an appointment with the Lloydys. With her tiny device inserted into my bits, Dave asked me, "Have you ever done it this way and was it good for you?" *Humour is what gets Dave and I through* those awkward moments, but maybe it was a little too much for her? Oh the look on the poor specialist's face, that memory still brings a smile to my face! *Laughter and humour* got us through so many of those tough, hideously embarrassing personal moments with medical professionals who we had never met before.

Look for the positives

Because I was traveling and needed to take so much medication, I had Dr Nick write me a letter just in case I was ever questioned at the airport. Well, that letter has done some extra trips for the charity just in case we were ever stopped by customs. We would often get near to use by date or damaged packets of items donated from pharmacies that were desperately needed by the programs we supported, but the volumes were sometimes a concern and we often wondered how strange the contents must have looked on the X-ray machine. Picture *10 litres of body wash* for sensitive baby skin in the bags of someone visiting for seven days! Or when Sue had her carry-on luggage full of old people's *Tena nappies.* I so wish she had been stopped that day and checked by customs. *Thirty nappies for an 8 hour flight!*

Customs can be pretty scary so I always felt safe with my trusty doctor's letter!

And one day I nearly needed to pull it out. I may not have told my sister and our friend how much had been donated by a local pharmacy, otherwise she would have worried. When we got to customs and my bag went through, the customs guy announced abruptly, "You have a lot of medicine." As I dug into my bag for my letter, Sue promptly stepped forward, having no idea how much medication was in there, and said it was for the children, the sick heart children. He responded with, "That's a lot of medicine for the sick children," but proceeded to let us through. If only you could have seen *Sue's face* when I showed her back at the hotel the 3,850 Ibuprofen in my bag!

See, some good can come from bad!

Being on the sideline

One thing about IVF is that you can have the most amazing people in your life, but it's so hard for them to truly understand what you are going through or say the right thing. Don't be too hard on them, find the right support and talk; *don't bottle it up.* As for those people that make you want to scream, stay away from them and only see them when you're not twitching and hypersensitive from all the drugs (FYI I'm already bawling my eyes out as Dave lies asleep next to me and I've finally decided to put pen to paper, or more accurately put index finger to iPhone about my journey). Where was I? Yes, it sucks, but *find people that can make you laugh* as you *share the hideous side effects!* Like my work colleagues, who share tweezers and a mirror with me just to keep those extra *chin hairs* under control.

Opinions - I'm *so Jack* of everyone's opinions on what I should and shouldn't do, and you can *stick your miracle stories* too!

What not to say

One of my gorgeous girlfriends told me once that she just *didn't know how to say the right thing* right now, and my response was, "the best thing you can do is just not even attempt to". Sometimes a *hug means so much more* than someone trying to find the right words, because the reality for me was that unless you could give me a baby, nothing you could say would make it better. That by far beats the shit out of things that can accidentally come tumbling out of your mouth. Don't get me wrong, I am sure I said some shockers to my friends that did IVF before me, trying to be helpful!

Some things to try to avoid from my own experience are:

It's so unfair I can just fall pregnant at the drop of a hat.
(Um, how does that help me feel anything but even more incapable/inadequate as a woman)

You can have my eggs. (Only say it if you really mean it)

I'll give you my husband's sperm. **(Maybe check what the problem is first before offering bodily fluids)**

My aunt's cousin's gardener miraculously fell pregnant after giving up on IVF for blah blah many years, you'll be right, it will happen. **(Again, know the problem before offering a miracle)**

Or the comment, *'don't worry good things come to those that wait'.* **Argh, no they effing don't! I remember getting that in a text from a friend that was preggers with her naturally conceived second baby and wanting to throw my phone off a bridge!**

Don't get me wrong, I had family and friends say some incredible things, write me beautiful text messages, give me huge hugs, wipe away my tears. But if you don't know what to say, that's perfectly okay, it means more just to know you care and that I'm in your thoughts.

What to say

I guess what I haven't written about is what to say when you are watching a loved one go through this incredibly tough journey. So, here are some of the beautiful messages I got from amazing family/friends that lifted my spirits and enabled me to stay positive and continue my fight. And a fight is exactly what it is, trying to stay positive and not letting the sadness win.

Hi Jen, just wanted to say thanks for yesterday. I had a great time, as always. I think you are amazing to have gone through such a tough year and then be so positive about the year ahead. I am crossing fingers and toes for a great year for you guys in 2016. You deserve it.

Looking forward to our next catch up xx

Please let me know when your book comes out, I want to be the first to buy a copy

Oh wrenny, I am so sorry, that is gut wrenching news for you both, it breaks my heart after all that you have been through. I can imagine there are no words right now! Sending big hugs your way. xxx

It is a horrible feeling to wake up to a reality that hurts every day and there isn't anything anyone can do or say to make it feel better. Finding the strength to face each day can be so hard. It is just shit! Thinking of you and sending you lots of love xxx

Hey Jen, was so good to see you yesterday. You looked beautiful... I know you probably won't be feeling it but you really did! Was great to catch up. Lloydie was absolutely hilarious... He is trouble!! You're lucky to have him and visa versa. Enjoy your break and hopefully some good downtime.

See you in the New Year! X

Share
(that's my recommendation)

One client told me that she didn't tell anyone at work during her journey, and that she regretted it because it was so hard to keep up appearances. I must admit I recruited for her during that time, unknowingly whilst she was on her journey, and I remember at times thinking that she was a bit flaky and never around. Well, I sure know why now. Trying to juggle specialist appointments, blood tests, ivig treatments, intralilip treatments is hugely challenging, but thanks to smart phones I did loads of work in medical waiting rooms.

What I also did was *share and share until we all cried* laughing in the office – having the girls check for out of control chin hair or just scaring them with too many details. Like the day I was convinced I'd found my colleague's future husband, and that I'd checked for a ring and looked him up on the Monash IVF site but if they were going to marry I'd have to have a chat with him first about the fact that he had had his face way tooooooooo close to my lady parts for an egg transfer!

OMG, I feel like *half of Australia has looked at my bits!* The first time I cried at the personal nature of the examinations, but by internal ultrasound number three I'd whipped my pants down whilst the ultrasound nurse was still in the room asking if I had any latex allergies, only to find out that she was the trainee and when the supervising nurse arrived we all laughed about how easy I was! Talk about getting your pants down quick!

Why can't we just talk about it?

Now, having grown up with a psychologist for a sister and knowing the sorts of clients she worked with, *I thought only really messed up people went to counselling.* When you think about it, they say losing a child is the hardest thing to do as a parent, but what about all of the IVF women/couples who see a tiny dot on an ultrasound but they lose the embryos time and time again? Now that's a grief that no one really talks about. It's no surprise that so many couples don't survive IVF, it's a grief that isn't really talked about or considered. You are just expected to take the failures, be compared to everyone's second cousin's aunt's work colleague who finally had success after 8 years, and push through!

Well news flash, *it ain't that effing easy!*

If you find yourself struggling with your grief and in need of professional support, don't be afraid to contact one of the wonderful IVF nurses, or a psychologist, and if it's during those long, lonely hours in the middle of the night, then please call a support line so that *you don't have to suffer alone.*

Lifeline – 13 1114   Beyond Blue – 1300 224 636

Changes

Your opinions and thoughts will change throughout this journey. There were things I didn't think I would do, but then the *IVF bar kept getting moved* and as the list of complications grew so did my thoughts on how far we would go.

What I thought I would never try or do or believe just kept changing, so if you had a set opinion on how long or what you would try, or even your thoughts on donor embryo/sperm or surrogacy, it's *okay if your opinion changes,* desperation does that to you. If I was talking to my former self from 3 years ago, I'm sure we would be having a discussion with very different opinions on what we would end up trying and how far we were prepared to go.

Be Thankful

Although I haven't been successful 'yet', words cannot describe the respect and admiration I have for Dr Nick and my amazing IVF nurses, Emily and Alex. I consider myself one of the lucky ones because Dr Nick is a 'no bullshit' kinda guy. He won't let you do endless rounds of IVF with no answers. He'll keep testing you and trying new ground-breaking medications, and he will tell you when enough is enough. And that's exactly what he did. As we went for our fifth egg collection he told me this was my last, because if it didn't work then it wasn't going to because I wasn't getting any younger. I replied with a smile, "If it wasn't for you I wouldn't feel so old, I would still feel like I'm 27!" We laughed and knew what our plan was. I'm *eternally grateful* for his brutal honesty, not letting me put my body through it again for nothing. I will always have the answers that some women don't ever get. So ladies, if you aren't getting the answers you need find a specialist that will keep conducting tests and trying something new. The definition of insanity is doing the same thing over and over again with the same outcome! At least I can say I even gave embryo glue a go – I don't think too many women can say that.

To Emily and Alex, you never ceased to amaze me with how much *generosity and kindness* you offered. I often thought how awful it must be to make yet another heartbreaking call to tell a patient that their blood test was negative. What amazing women! I don't think words can truly sum up what you both did for me at different times, *thank you xx*

And to all the Monash team, you ladies are great, especially the pre-op nurses who are like angels. Possibly the only highlight was the few seconds between the injection and being put to sleep for another procedure. What a happy place, one of the nurses patting your hand, smiling and comforting you.

Don't forget to thank people along your journey. Think about it from their side. It can't be much fun at times in their roles, delivering heartbreaking news and being on the end of those IVF moods. Oh, and don't chew out the accounts ladies, they are simply doing their job! They too think it's huge sums of money you are paying, but it sure as hell is out of their control.

Dr Maz kept me sane

I'll be honest in saying that I didn't know a lot about Chinese medicine or what it could do, but I'd known Maz since my early 20s and it'd been a few years when I saw her at my brother's birthday party. Well, she looked amazing, I swear she hadn't aged a bit, and my sister-in-law told me she was a *qualified Chinese doctor*, with an amazing way of eating and living. I thought I had better get onto this stuff so I could look amazing again too! So I marched myself down to see her the very next week. At the time I was bloated beyond belief and feeling a number of side effects. Now don't get me wrong, I hate the Chinese herbs and hold my nose to get through them, many a time cooking them up and just looking at them, but between the potions and acupuncture she made the process so much easier. I don't think I could have got through it without her.

I remember the day I went to see Dr Maz and she hadn't asked me a question or done any consultation, she simply looked at me and said, "You are having trouble seeing aren't you?" She could just tell by looking at my contorted face. I'd not said much to anyone and had been trying to power through at work, and maybe I drove with just one eye open to focus! Why did I do this? Because if you had blurred vision as a side effect you were to stop taking the medication and I was desperate for it to work and not to give up! I was definitely at the point of thinking the meds had won and I couldn't take it anymore, but *Dr Maz kept me sane* and did amazing work to relieve the side effects. I'll always be very grateful as she got many a tear, handed me the tissues, reminded me that what I was putting my body and mind through was so tough and that I was doing so well under the circumstances. I placed all of my faith in modern medicine, but I was also open to alternative treatments and have no doubt that they have worked together to keep my body and my mind strong enough to get through all of this. Thanks for always being there for me, Dr Maz!

SOME WORDS FROM DR MAZ

In Chinese Medicine, we understand that each person is unique, and what helps to bring balance and wellbeing to one person's system may do the opposite for someone else. A very basic example can be seen in how hot, dry weather helps some people feel more comfortable (i.e. many people with joint pain or arthritis) while others may experience an exacerbation of existing symptoms (i.e. hayfever, skin rashes, headaches).

Likewise, each person's journey towards parenthood is also highly individual. Though there are often common side effects that many will experience, each individual will respond in their own unique way, and what helps one person feel better on their IVF journey might not do much for another – some people find they need more quiet time at rest to support the changes in their system, while others might feel more balanced for incorporating regular movement to help their body process everything that's going on.

This is why it's important to:

BE KIND AND GENTLE WITH YOURSELF
You are doing amazing things every day! You might not feel like fitting in all the things that you normally do in your life, and that's ok.

TAKE TIME TO BE STILL AND LISTEN TO YOURSELF, and HONOUR WHAT YOU NEED
(This will likely change from day to day, and that's ok). You know best what you need in each moment: we all have this ability, but sometimes life gets so busy that we don't have time in to tune into ourselves. Taking 10 minutes each day in silence, without distractions, to focus on your breath will help you hear what you need. This can be seated, lying down, or even as a walking meditation.

ASK FOR HELP IF YOU NEED IT
One of the million reasons why this book is so amazing is that it can help the people around you understand what you are going through, and I'm sure many of these people would love to help if asked.

SOME GENERAL CHINESE MEDICINE HEALTH TIPS

The schedules, medications and expectations that come with IVF can put a lot of stress on the mind and body, so it's helpful to lighten the overall load on your system with the following:

SLEEP

Contemporary research now confirms what Chinese Medicine has advised for millennia – adequate sleep is essential for good health, and particularly so when your system is taking on the added workload or assimilating medications. Aim for 7-8 hours nightly, and avoid screens and bright lights for at least an hour before bed. Our system do a lot of their daily clean-up between 10pm and 2am, so aim to be asleep by 10pm to reap maximum benefits.

COOKED FOODS, WARM DRINKS

In Chinese Medicine we focus on cooked foods, which are easier to digest, resulting in better assimilation of nutrients and less bloating and other discomforts. Similarly, warm drinks keep the digestive system ticking over nicely – anyone who has experienced an ice-cream headache has experienced a strong message from the belly that it doesn't love the cold!

AND AVOID MULTI-TASKING WHEN EATING

Trying to work (or being distracted by screens or information overload) while eating diverts the necessary energy away from the digestive organs. I always remind my patients of this, and encourage them to take a few minutes before eating for some restorative, deep, belly breaths: this signals to the body that it is ok to drop into "rest and digest" mode, and focus on digesting and assimilating nutrients.

KEEP YOUR FEET WARM, DON'T WALK BAREFOOT ON COLD TILES, etc.
(barefoot beachwalks are great though!)

The acupuncture channels / muscle chains that wrap around the reproductive organs have their origin in the feet. Freezing the feet will slow down the flow of blood and lymph along this whole pathway – the opposite of what we are trying to achieve when boosting reproductive health. So keep those feet warm – Epsom salt foot baths are a great way to do this, and contain Magnesium to calm the nervous system as an added bonus. Try them before bed for awesome sleep!

PROTECT YOUR NECK AND SHOULDERS

Acupuncturists are notorious for reminding their patients to wrap up against drafts / open car windows / air-conditioning in order to protect against colds! It helps keep bugs at bay, which is very helpful when you might already be battling side-effects of meds, or feeling low on energy.

TAKE TIME OUT FOR YOU

Our culture glorifies being busy, multi-tasking and achievement, but busy times need quiet times (doing "nothing") to balance them out. The added benefit of taking quiet time is that calming your nervous system can have a beneficial effect on your hormones too! Even a few minutes of slow, deep breathing can break the stress response and that running-on-adrenaline feeling. So, lie down, pop your feet up, and rest your hands on your lower belly. Allow the breath to fill up the belly before it fills up the chest – you can let the rise and fall of your hands be an indicator of how deeply you're breathing. Focus on the exhale – making it longer than the inhale is another way of giving your nervous system the message that's its ok to calm down and let go. Do this as many times during the day as you like, even sitting at work / clinic / on the train, etc. I also love the "Triangle Breath": see below.

ACUPUNCTURE & CHINESE MEDICINE (OBVIOUSLY!!)

This is a powerful treatment for rebalancing the nervous system. Repeated studies have shown that acupuncture can promote relaxation and reduce stress. It is also a wonderful modality that integrates well with IVF treatment and can ease its associated side effects, without adding more drugs to the mix.

balancedacupuncture.com.au

1   Eshkevari, L., Egan, R., Phillips, D., Tilan, J., Carney, E., Azzam, N., Amri, H. & Mulroney, S. E. (2012). Acupuncture at ST36 prevents chronic stress-induced increases in neuropeptide Y in rat. Experimental Biology and Medicine; vol. 237 no. 1, pp. 18-23.

Eshkevari, L., Permaul, E. & Mulroney, S. E. (2013) Acupuncture blocks cold stress-induced increases in the hypothalamus–pituitary–adrenal axis in the rat. Journal of Endocrinology; vol. 217, pp. 95-104.

Hollifield, M., Sinclair-Lian, N., Warner, T. D. & Hammerschlag, R. (2007). Acupuncture for Posttraumatic Stress Disorder: A Randomized Controlled Pilot Trial. Journal of Nervous & Mental Disease, vol. 195 no. 6, pp. 504-513.

Kim, H., Park, H., Han, S., Hahn, D., Lee, H., Kim, K. & Shim, I. (2009). The effects of acupuncture stimulation at PC6 (Neiguan) on chronic mild stress-induced biochemical and behavioral responses. Neuroscience Letters, vol. 460 no. 1, pp.56-60.

Schroeder, S., Burnis, J., Denton, A., Krasnow, A., Raghu, T. S. & Mathis, K. (2017). Effectiveness of Acupuncture Therapy on Stress in a Large Urban College Population. Journal of Acupuncture and Meridian Studies; vol. 10 no. 3, pp.165-170.

TRIANGLE BREATH

Shallow, rapid breaths are a message to the body that it should be prepared for fight or flight. They can perpetuate adrenaline release and keep us in high-alert mode, even once stress or danger has passed. Conversely, breathing slowly, deeply and mindfully encourages the body to feel safe. A particularly effective way of signaling safety to the nervous system is by extending the length of your exhalation (in a dangerous situation, you wouldn't have time to leisurely and completely empty your lungs!). This wonderfully simple exercise uses the concept of a triangle to regulate your in- and out- breaths.

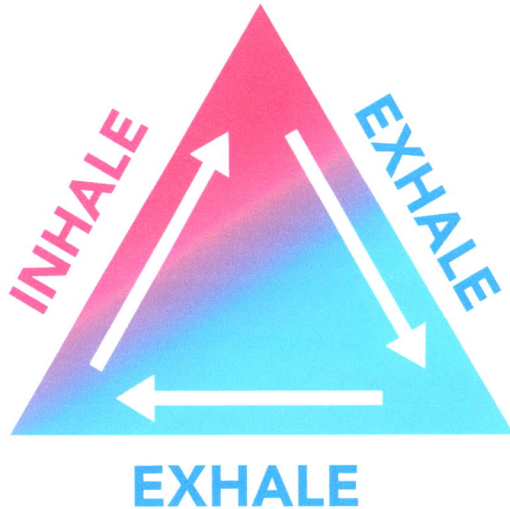

1. *Sit or lay comfortably (preferably with a straight spine)*

2. *Take a few moments to allow your breath to settle into its natural rhythm, and note how long each inhale and exhale lasts (for most people this is somewhere between 3 and 6 counts).*

3. *The idea now is to lengthen the exhale so it is roughly twice as long as your inhale. So, using our triangle below, we inhale for the length of one side (for example, a count of 3), and then exhale for the length of the two remaining sides (3 + 3), drawing the exhale out nice and long. Keep the breathing gentle: don't force the breath, and if you find you are running out of exhale, it's absolutely ok to shorten the count - just keep the inhale longer than the exhale. As your body relaxes, you may find that your inhales and exhales get naturally slower.*

4. *Once you return to the beginning point on the triangle, start again. Aim for a few minutes of triangle breathing as a daily practice, or whenever you are feeling the need to reduce stress.*

Final words of advice

The final thing I will say is this – you may agree with what worked for me and maybe you won't, and there is *nothing wrong with that.* Find out what makes the hell days of waiting for results and the pain easier for you, and whatever that is, enjoy! The series 'Suits' on Netflix certainly helped take my mind off things. Dave and I would have couch time series sessions whilst we were waiting for the phone to ring with blood test results. Seeing Mike Ross and Harvey Specter always managed to distract me!

For those support people, family and friends – hopefully you've *giggled, shed a tear,* thought about what you've said and found a better way to respond from reading this book. But if you still can't keep your foot out of your mouth, *flowers always work!*

May your journey bring you the bundle of joy your heart so desires.

TIPS

It's probably important to tell you...

Tip No 1:

Always carry tweezers! There is nothing wrong with having them hidden everywhere. Don't leave home without them, because those extra hairs feel like they come up in seconds! You are never safe from one!

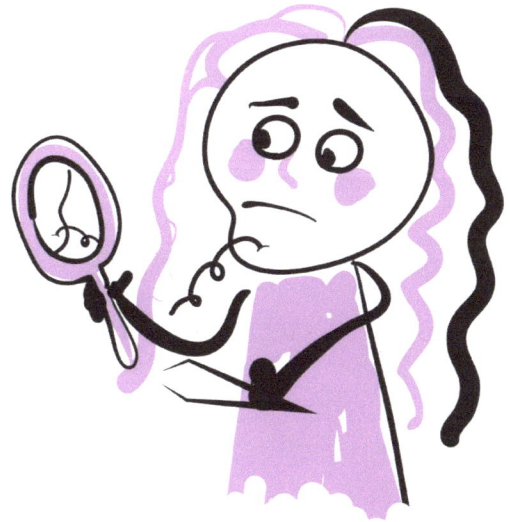

Tip No 2:

TISSUES. During IVF, apparently I became a nanna, as a younger friend told me only nannas carry those special little pre-packed, neatly folded, purse-size Kleenex tissue packs. Buy them in bulk and hide them wherever you can too! Why? Because some of those drugs make you cry non-stop. One Saturday in my first year of IVF I was reading Anh Doh's book, *The Happiest Refugee*. It wasn't during the sad part, I was actually laughing out aloud at his brother being mistaken for a girl by the Salvos and wearing girl's clothes for the first year or two he was in Australia (if you haven't read it I would highly recommend you do). Anyway, there I was laughing and crying hysterically for no reason. Watch out for those tears, they sneak up on you and just when you think you can cry no more, out come more tears and more snot, which leads me to a question. Where does it come from? Surely I should lose weight with all that excess water loss! Unfortunately not.

Tip No 3:

In the words of my incredible Chinese Doctor Maz – *be kind to yourself.* What do I mean by that? What you are doing to yourself is torture, both physically and mentally, and that doesn't even touch on the financial burden. If you only manage to get up, find clothes that fit and get through the day, you've done well. Don't push yourself to be the energetic, upbeat, laugh-a-minute kinda girl you normally are when just breathing and holding it together deserves a medal!

Tip No 4:

Happy pants. Yep you heard me, those MC Hammer pants from the 80s are a necessity! Whilst on a trip to Vietnam I purchased three pairs because I thought they would be comfy in the heat. Well, it turns out that they also work wonders on those days when you've done so many injections that you are bloated beyond belief, when 4kgs of fluid pile on in just a few days. That's right, ladies, happy pants are a girl's best friend! Um, and yes I still wear them most days as I start to kick the kilos that I've piled on!

Tip No 5:

A dear friend of happy pants is Havaianas – yep that's right! Flowing pants and thongs (jandals for my kiwi friends) were great on those fluid filled days when your favourite three-inch high heels just don't fit like they used to anymore for some strange reason, as your cankles hang over the top. Don't worry, they do go back to their original size... eventually!

Cankles

When the calves and feet are connecting showing no ankle. It's extremely NASTY.[2]

2   Urban Dictionary

My Emotions

Everyone Hurts

To the women going through IVF – although this process is agony for you, don't forget that those around you feel your pain and are hurting too. My parents were desperate to be grandparents again, and seeing their sadness reminded me that they were hurting too. To my amazing sister, brother and sister-in-law that have adopted my step children as their own, I so wish I could give them the joy of being an Aunty or Uncle to my children, as I know from the joy I get when I am with my nephew and niece what a truly amazing feeling it is! And to Dave, my desire to give you another little Lloydy... there are no words to describe.

Devastation

The day I found out I would never look into the eyes of my child and see myself was the hardest day. Why is my body so cruel?? We were told it was highly unlikely the transfer would work, but what option did we have? We did the transfer and I felt so different this time around. My period didn't come before the blood test, so even though we knew it was such a slim chance, in that last 48 hours I'd really started to believe it had worked! I'd started planning how I would tell people, the conversation I'd have with my boss about going part-time, and then bang, it failed! Talk about coming crashing back down to reality, a reality that I would never look into the eyes of my child and see myself! A reality that sucks my breath away every time I think about it.

No *New Idea* or *Women's Weekly* miracle baby front cover here. My eggs were simply too old, their quality too poor, and it was not going to work.

Depression

On the day I found out it didn't work for the final time with my own egg, I went to pick up our favourite take away for dinner in a daze. It was like my body was on autopilot, one foot in front of the other and no one was home upstairs. As I stood at the boom gate waiting for the passing train there was a moment, a brief moment where I wondered, if I stepped out in front of the train what the initial impact would feel like. Would I just feel like I was floating, would the aching pain in my chest be gone? Now, I would never have done it because I couldn't do it to my Dave, family and friends, but especially not my sister because she had already lost too much. But the drugs that I was on did have the side effect of depression and anxiety, plus about another 45 side effects, and although I knew I was deeply sad it was those hideous steroids that let me think that way. They were promptly thrown in the bin, and I went cold turkey (which you aren't supposed to do) and got that crap out of my system so I could function and process my grief properly.

I now have a deep appreciation for those that struggle with mental health and depression, because that day gave me an insight into what their daily struggles must feel like. My heart breaks for you.

Remember ladies, when you are having those dark moments, and I'll be honest that wasn't the only time I wondered what sweet relief from the pain would feel like, remember the old you is still inside but the drugs are talking and some days they just aren't your friend. So hold tight, things will get better and you will get back to being able to smell the roses, it will just take time.

And if you don't trust that you can beat the voices in your head, reach out and let someone know that today it's just too hard for you to do it alone.

My final words from my heart...

2.30am Friday 6th November 2015

As I write this I still haven't made my decision, but of course I know deep down that despite the very low chance of success, I'll implant the one frosty I have in the lab and hope like hell it sticks. But beyond that, can I consider alternatives? It's interesting how flippantly people suggest surrogacy and adoption. To them it seems so easy; you should just do it if you REALLY want children. Unless you are staring down the barrel of those things being your only options, you never truly know what you'll consider or do. Over the years, and as the journey has gotten harder, my thoughts and opinions have changed. What I do know is that no one has the right to judge you, or in fact have an opinion on what you choose to do, because no one can truly understand your heartache and devastation at one failed attempt after the next. Whatever you choose, be kind to yourself over the process and whatever your loved one/s choose, all you can be is their rock and hug them tight because it's just simply something you cannot understand and it's okay not to. IVF is just so damn complex and personal. As I have said before, your journey is yours and no two journeys are the same. I wonder whether by the time I finish this book I will know all the answers, or maybe I will be ready to write a follow up book!

6.40am Monday 14th December 2015

So three days after my world crashed down around me, my Christmas party, which I've been hosting for 16 years, was upon me. There were bucket-loads of champagne, I was doing so well and then bang, there I was bawling again. But I was lucky enough to be surrounded by all of my favourite people. Needless to say, eight days later, I haven't had a day without tears! Surely that will come soon. And every morning I wake up thinking, 'what drug do I need to take today?' – it's like ground hog day as I have that sharp pain in my chest and realisation that my dream is over and the only silver lining is I don't need to do a pessary before work!

Where to next? I'm not sure. My pincushion body needs a break, my wallet is empty, I'm still a little bit twitchy from coming off all the drugs, but I still hope and pray that I'll get to be a mum one day. For now it's Christmas with those I love and my amazing step-children.

4.54am Monday 21st December 2015

I can't sleep and that ache in my chest just won't go away. I realise that I've been on some form of medication for most of the last 3 years, with a maximum break of 6 weeks, and I simply don't know what to do. I almost feel like I'm lost without counting days in my diary. What was my life like before IVF? Struggling to adjust to a normal non-IVF life and simply being me, being able to plan and commit to social events, and to relax and not worry about dates and times – how bizarre!

My incredible step-children are down from Sydney for Christmas, and as we sat on the couch, all four of us laughing, mucking around and watching TV, I wondered to myself, could this be enough, could I end my IVF journey here?

Xx Jen

Thursday 25th February 2016

It's funny how I've been on this journey for nearly 3 years and I could put so much down on the iPhone in a couple of days, and then I have moments when I just want to be normal and forget, and can't even bring myself to read what I have written. I'm yet to be able to read what I have written over the past months without bursting into tears. I'm trying to get this mind dump to a point that an editor can look at it but I just can't get through it, so luckily my sister has offered to put it into a more understandable order and not just my jumbled middle-of-the-night thoughts!

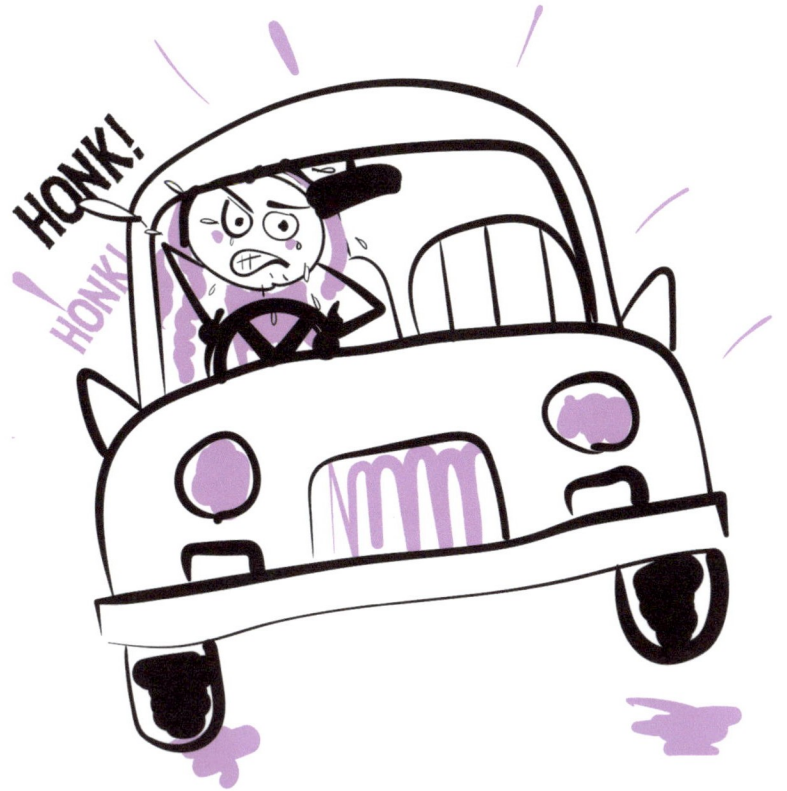

What did I learn from this journey?

I've always been fiercely protective and loyal (my sister Sue sure can tell a story or two about that) but I probably didn't protect myself enough. What I have definitely learnt from this is to put myself first, stand up for myself, speak my mind and stand by the things I've said and done. I don't really know why, but somehow through all of this I've gained confidence I never had!

I've always considered myself an eternal optimist. This journey has broken me at times, but I've come out still the eternal optimist who has bad days and still cries but that's okay, life isn't fair sometimes. I've probably spent more nights drunk than I have sober in the last couple of weeks but I'm back, I'm kicking 2015 to the curb, I'm going to get my pre IVF body back! Because that's probably been one of the hardest things, buying sizes of clothes that I never thought I ever would, and sadly not maternity ones. 2016 and I are going to be the best of friends, all good things come to those who wait. Right? Well I've waited and now I'm ready for good things in 2016!

May my story bring you some solace in knowing you're not alone! I'm right beside you, ready to wipe away those tears. May your journey bring you happiness and the bundle of joy your heart so desires. Xx

Epilogue

August 2017

Yesterday morning I woke up and my first thought was that I needed to finish this book and now. I haven't been able to write anything for 18 months and have barely been able to read what I had already written, which is why it's still sitting here, waiting for me to feel brave enough to tackle the final edit! But yesterday the decision was made and I knew I needed to do it. I feel like the time is right, as that very same morning I headed to a networking breakfast to see Gail Kelly (former Westpac CEO) speak about the book she had launched, and I met up with my gorgeous friend, Steph Woollard. She gave me a copy of her newly released book, 'From a Tin Shed to the United Nations'. I took these 'book moments' as a sign and knew that I had to finish what I had started. I mentioned to Steph that I was going to Greece for 'one last crack' and she said it'd be a great name for a book, or at least a chapter!

Then only 5 days later I saw my sister and mentioned my weird, overwhelming 'must do' thoughts about the book, and she told me she had also had a weird dream and had been thinking for a week that we must finish the book before I made the journey to Greece. So here I am, back on my iPhone while Dave sleeps, planning the final bits of the book, while Sue is spending the weekend doing the final edits (this is because some of it is so raw and painful that I just can't read it and her ability to turn my thoughts and notes into something more readable
is amazing).

One Last Crack!

So here I am, up to my eyeballs in drugs, so many in a day that I need to write a schedule that's stuck on the fridge where I tick them off!

This is my current daily schedule:

2 x Megafol as soon as I wake up
2 x Dexamethasone with brekkie
1 x Asprin with brekkie
1 x Progynova with brekkie
9.30am Synard nasal spray
1 x Progynova with lunch
1 x multivitamin
1 x Progynova with dinner
9.30pm Synard nasal spray
Day done and off to bed!

Next week I have to add more drugs and injections and pessaries (any ladies that have ever had to have the 'rockets' knows how damn awful they are) to the list!

This is it, we are going as far as I'm prepared to go with IVF. I'm nervous that I still won't pass the remaining tests but I am staying as brave and positive as I can and trying to think good thoughts. We are off overseas next week in search of success! Wish us luck, I hope that the end of this long nightmare of a journey will be the good news story we have dreamed of for 5 years now – it will be our only good news story in all of these years of IVF! I can only hope. Xx

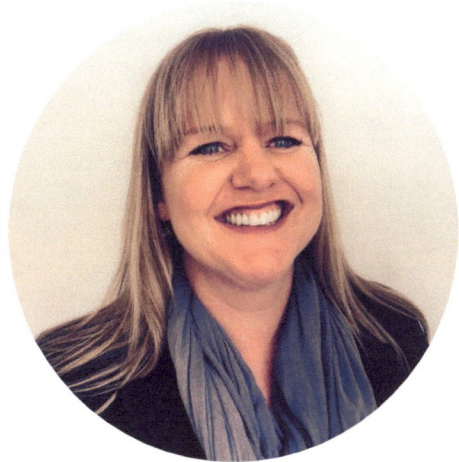

Jenny Lloyd

Jenny Lloyd is a business owner and writer, and has drawn on her own experiences to tell a raw personal journey and sometimes bleakly funny story on a subject that is not often discussed outwardly. Not only does she successfully run her own company, *Lloyd Connect*, but along with her sister, she co-founded *Helping Hand Helping Hearts*. Among other initiatives, the charitable organisation assists children in Vietnam to receive life-saving heart surgery, as well as funding a shelter for pregnant mothers and helping to support a charity school.

Jenny loves to travel and is a keen cook, who gains great pleasure from sharing a meal she has created with her family and friends.

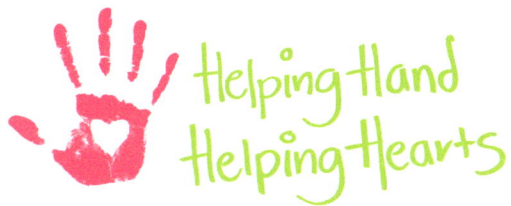

Helping Hand Helping Hearts

10% of all proceeds from the sale of this book will go to *Helping Hand Helping Hearts*, a charitable foundation my sister and I set up in memory of her late husband Nick, who passed away from heart disease at the age of 40.

HHHH is my proudest achievement yet, and we have just funded our 100th heart surgery in Vietnam for underprivileged children in partnership with Heartbeat Vietnam. 100% of all donations go directly to our beneficiaries, something Sue and I are very proud of as we self-fund all administration costs. I'm very pleased to be able to use sales from this book to continue our incredible work.

www.hhhh.org.au

Thank you

Where do I start? Firstly, thank you to my gorgeous friend Lawrence, who told me that my take on IVF was so funny that I should write a book. Well, I took on your advice and here it is!

To Dave, my partner in crime, thank you for everything, what a ride it has been! Thanks for picking me back up and loving me no matter what.

To Sue, my older and wiser but petite big sister, without your support and editing skills through all of this, the book would still be in notes on my iPhone. Thank you for believing in me.

To Amber, what can I say except that you got it. You always managed to send the best texts and you and Mac did such an incredible job of picking me back up and always having me drop in for cuddles with my precious niece and nephew on those awful days.

Mum and Dad, your support has been endless!

Dr Maz, my rock...I have so much appreciation for your work, friendship and bedside manner!

To some of my old work colleagues, thanks for laughing with me through the crazy IVF side effects and letting me know when I had out of control chin hair. Sri Sri, you were the best for letting me use your tweezers in those emergency moments.

There are so many other people I am grateful to, you know who you are! So thank you for your help on this journey so far xx

Reflections

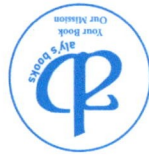

www.ingramcontent.com/pod-product-compliance
Lightning Source LLC
Chambersburg PA
CBHW040929030426
42334CB00002B/19